Homemade Foot Spa

48 All Natural Foot Soak
Foot Scrubs, Foot Creams &
Heel Balms for Tired Feet,
Dry Skin, Foot Odor & Other
Foot Problems

Table of Contents

	Page
Introduction	1a
Benefits of Good Foot Care	1
Beware of Products Containing Hidden Toxins	3
Foot Scrubs Introduction	5
Soothing Tea Tree Foot Scrub	6
Muscovado Foot Scrub	7
Simple Peppermint Foot Scrub	8
Papaya Foot Scrub	9
Pumpkin Foot Scrub	10
Simple Strawberry Foot Scrub	11
Choco Foot Scrub	12
Caribbean Spa Foot Scrub	13
Buttery Banana Foot Scrub	14
Lively Lemongrass Foot Scrub	15
Epsom Salt Foot Scrub	16
Coconut Lime Foot Scrub	17
Coffee Foot Scrub	18
Peanut Lemon Foot Scrub	19
Avocado Foot Scrub	20
Foot Soaks Introduction	21
Minty Lime Foot Soak	22
Lemon Foot Odor Soak	23
Magnificent Milk & Honey Foot Soak	24
Luscious Lavender Foot Soak	25
Rice Foot Soak	26
Really Rosy Foot Soak	27
Emergency Foot Reviver	28
Calming Chamomile Foot Soak	29
Olive Lemon Foot Soak	30
Orange Foot Soak	31

Apple Cider Vinegar Foot Soak   32
Easy Eucalyptus Foot Soak   33
Forget Fungus Foot Soak   34
Aching Feet Foot Soak   35
Super Sore Foot Soak   36
Orange & Ginger Foot Soak   37
Dead Sea Salts Soak   38
Jasmine Foot Soak   39
Pumpkin Foot Soak   40
Grapefruit Foot Soak   41
Smelly Feet Foot Soak   42
Tired Feet Foot Soak   43
Sweet Cucumber Foot Soak   44
Heel Balms Introduction   45
Rich Coco Heel Balm   46
Cinnamon & Orange Heel Balm   47
Neem Heel Balm   48
Jojoba Heel Balm   49
Emu Oil Heel Balm   50
Lavender Heel Balm   51
Honey Orange Heel Balm   52
Organic Olive Oil Heel Balm   53
Shea & Lemongrass Heel Balm   54
Tea Tree Heel Balm   55
Conclusion   56
My Other Homemade Beauty Product Books 56

Introduction

Hello and welcome,

In this book, I am giving you **48** of my best **Homemade Foot Scrubs, Foot Soaks, Foot Creams & Heel Balm Recipes.**

What makes all these recipes fabulous is how quickly you can put them together. Once you have bought a few basic ingredients then you will be able to make lots of these soothing foot products not only for you and your family, but for your friends and colleagues too. There's a good chance that you already have many of the ingredients needed to create these products at home.

There is nothing better than treating your feet. They are one of the most used parts of our bodies so we need to pay maximum attention to looking after them. What you put on your skin is ever so important as well. When you make your own foot care treatments, you know **EXACTLY** what is in them and you can alter any recipe to suit yourself. No more unhealthy and dangerous products for you. Natural all the way!

The sky is the limit when it comes to making your own natural foot treatment products. You are only limited by your own imagination. Anything is possible. Are you ready to pamper your feet?

Lorraine xx

Benefits of Good Foot Care

Foot care and massage has been practiced for centuries in many cultures as a way of healing illnesses, relieving stress and helping to ease tired and aching feet. In today's society, we don't prioritise as much time to look after our feet as well as we should.

We tend to pay lots of attention to our hands, face and body but we often neglect our feet. With everything form ill-fitting shoes to bunions and corns, our feet are taking a right battering these days.

Taking regular footbaths to help relieve the aches and pains of the day, for reviving your tired feet and for pampering purposes should be the norm, not the exception.

A bit of a rest and a nice warm foot bath cab really help to take the stresses of the day away, help increase blood circulation and help to decrease joint pains.

Notes About Your Foot Care & The Recipes In This Book

- Use good quality oils and butters to nourish your skin and feed it with the best nutrients. The salts used in these recipes help to clean, exfoliate and relax your feet so make sure you always have a supply to hand.
- Feel free to mix and match the oils and herbs used based on your favorite fragrances but don't forget that different herbs and oils offer different therapeutic benefits. You can treat a variety of foot problems with all the herbs and oils that nature provides for us so experiment and see what works best for you.
- Add marbles to the bottom of your basin or foot spa for a bit of extra luxury and massage for your feet.

Beware of Store Bought Products Containing Hidden Toxins

It was five years ago almost to the day that I decided to **STOP** putting harsh chemicals on my skin. This was after I researched the harmful and toxic ingredients that beauty product manufacturers put in our products.

They do this as a money saving exercise mainly and seem to show little if any concern for the end consumer. This made me angry!

The more I looked into the situation, the more I found out about how these toxins silently seep into your system through your skin. You might think "well I'm only putting these creams on my feet" but that doesn't matter. They can still be harmful.

Some of the nasty 'hidden' ingredients in some of my lotions and creams were:

- Synthetic (un-natural) fragrances
- Methlyparaben
- Oxybenzone
- Stearalkonium Chloride
- Diethanolamine
- Propylene Glycol
- Artificial colors

This is just a few that I can remember. When you look these ingredients up on the internet, like me, you will be horrified and surprised that these manufacturers get away with it. They not only get away with it, they actually make millions of dollars selling us all potentially harmful and poisonous products.

Rather than accept my toxic fate, I decided to take my health and beauty matters into my own hands and create my own products. I am proud to say that I haven't bought a shop bought beauty product for my face, body or feet in the last 5 years and I look and feel better than ever.

Conduct your own research and come to your own conclusions. I would guess though that as soon as you start looking into the harmful chemicals in your products yourself, like me you will abandon these store bought toxic mixtures and start making your own beauty products from the comfort of your home. You have to pay attention to the other parts of your body as well.

Are you ready to create the most simple and easy foot treatment recipes? Yes, well then let's get started!

Foot Scrubs

These foot scrubs are healing and moisturizing and extremely good for your feet. Pamper your feet with this collection of easy to make recipes. There's something for every mood so try them all, you will love them.

If the scrubs seem a little too dry for you simply add more oils. If the mixture is a little too wet then add more salt or sugar to your recipe. Make sure you sterilize your jars and/or containers before storing your scrubs, soaks and creams

Soothing Tea Tree Foot Scrub

Ingredients

- ½ cup sea salt
- ¼ cup almond oil
- 5 drops tea tree essential oil

Directions

1. In a bowl, mix all the ingredients together until well combined
2. Apply to feet and scrub gently
3. Allow the scrub to stay on your feet for at least 10 minutes
4. Rinse off and pat your feet dry
5. Apply your favorite moisturizer and enjoy your refreshed and soothed skin

Muscovado Foot Scrub

Ingredients

- ½ cup Muscovado sugar
- ¼ cup olive oil
- ¼ cup baking soda
- 3 drops tea tree essential oil

Directions

1. In a bowl, mix all the ingredients together until well combined
2. Apply to feet and scrub gently
3. Allow the scrub to stay on your feet for at least 10 minutes
4. Rinse off and pat your feet dry
5. Apply your favorite moisturizer and enjoy your beautiful skin

Simple Peppermint Foot Scrub

Ingredients

- ¼ cup sea salt
- 1 tablespoon olive oil
- 1 teaspoon coconut oil
- 3 drops peppermint essential oil
- 2 drops rosemary essential oil

Directions

1. In a bowl, mix all the ingredients together until well combined
2. Apply to feet and scrub gently
3. Allow the scrub to stay on your feet for at least 10 minutes (longer if you have time)
4. Rinse off and pat your feet dry
5. Apply your favorite moisturizer, your feet will feel great

Papaya Foot Scrub

Ingredients

- 1/8 cup Bora Bora White Sand
- 1/8 cup Kosher salt
- ½ teaspoon papaya fragrance oil
- ¼ cup papaya oil
- 3 drops tea tree essential oil
- 2 drops rose essential oil

Directions

1. In a bowl, mix all the ingredients together until well combined
2. Apply to feet and scrub gently
3. Allow the scrub to stay on your feet for at least 15 minutes
4. Rinse off and pat your feet dry
5. Apply your favorite moisturizer and enjoy your beautiful skin

Pumpkin Foot Scrub

Ingredients

- 1/8 cup white sugar
- 1/8 cup brown sugar
- 1/8 cup almond oil
- ½ cup fresh pumpkin
- 1 teaspoon cinnamon

Directions

1. In a bowl, mash the pumpkin until it is smooth
2. Add all the other ingredients and combine together
3. Apply to feet and scrub gently
4. Allow the scrub to stay on your feet for at least 10 minutes
5. Rinse off and pat your feet dry
6. Apply your favorite moisturizer and enjoy your lovely feet

Simple Strawberry Foot Scrub

Ingredients

- 4 strawberries
- 2 tablespoons grapeseed oil
- ¼ cup sea salt

Directions

1. In a bowl combine all the ingredients together
2. Apply to feet and scrub gently
3. Allow the scrub to stay on your feet for at least 10 minutes
4. Rinse off and dry your feet
5. Apply your favorite moisturizer and enjoy your lovely feet

Choco Foot Scrub

Ingredients

- ¼ cup brown sugar
- ¼ cup sea salt
- 1/8 cup olive oil
- 1/8 cup jojoba oil
- 2 tablespoons cocoa powder
- ½ teaspoon nutmeg
- ½ teaspoon cinnamon

Directions

1. In a bowl combine all the ingredients together
2. Apply to feet and scrub gently
3. Allow the scrub to stay on your feet for at least 10 minutes
4. Rinse off and dry your feet
5. Apply your favorite moisturizer and enjoy your renewed feet

Caribbean Spa Foot Scrub

Ingredients

- ¼ cup sea salt
- 1/8 cup olive oil
- 2 tablespoons fresh coconut (grated)
- 2 drops coconut essential oil
- 2 drops orange essential oil

Directions

1. In a bowl combine all the ingredients together
2. Apply to feet and scrub gently
3. Allow the scrub to stay on your feet for at least 15 minutes
4. Rinse off and pat dry your feet
5. Apply your favorite moisturizer and enjoy your lovely feet

Buttery Banana Foot Scrub

Ingredients

- 1 ripe banana
- 2 tablespoons sea salt
- 2 tablespoons olive oil
- 2 drops lemon essential oil

Directions

1. In a bowl mash the bananas a little
2. Mix in all the other ingredients in and blend it all together
3. Apply to feet and scrub gently
4. Allow the scrub to stay on your feet for at least 10 minutes
5. Rinse off and dry your feet
6. Apply your favorite moisturizer and enjoy your lovely feet

Lively Lemongrass Foot Scrub

Ingredients

- ¼ cup sea salt
- ¼ cup white sugar
- 2 tablespoons lemon grass fragrance oil
- 2 tablespoons grapeseed oil
- Pinch of fresh lemongrass

Directions

1. In a bowl combine all the ingredients together
2. Apply to feet and scrub gently
3. Allow the scrub to stay on your feet for at least 10 minutes
4. Rinse off and dry your feet
5. Apply your favorite moisturizer and enjoy your soft smooth skin

Epsom Salt Foot Scrub

Ingredients

- ½ cup Epsom salts
- ¼ cup olive oil
- 4 drops lavender essential oil

Directions

1. In a bowl combine all the ingredients together
2. Apply to feet and scrub gently
3. Allow the scrub to stay on your feet for at least 10 minutes
4. Rinse off and dry your feet
5. Apply your favorite moisturizer and enjoy your revitalized feet

Coconut & Lime Foot Scrub

Ingredients

- ½ cup brown sugar
- 2 tablespoons coconut oil
- 1 tablespoon grated lime peel

Directions

1. In a bowl combine all the ingredients together
2. Apply to feet and scrub gently
3. Allow the scrub to stay on your feet for at least 10 minutes (longer if you have time)
4. Rinse off and dry your feet
5. Apply your favorite moisturizer and enjoy your lovely feet

Coffee Foot Scrub

Ingredients

- ½ cup ground coffee
- 2 tablespoons coconut oil

Directions

1. In a bowl combine all the ingredients together
2. Apply to feet and scrub gently
3. Allow the scrub to stay on your feet for at least 15 minutes (longer if you have time)
4. Rinse off and dry your feet
5. Apply your favorite moisturizer and enjoy your revitalized feet

Peanut Lemon Foot Scrub

Ingredients

- ½ cup sea salt
- ¼ cup ground almonds
- 3 tablespoons olive oil
- 3 drops lemon essential oil
- 2 teaspoons fresh lemon juice

Directions

1. In a bowl combine all the ingredients together
2. Apply to feet and scrub gently
3. Allow the scrub to stay on your feet for 3-4 minutes
4. Rinse off and dry your feet
5. Apply your favorite moisturizer and enjoy your lovely feet

Avocado Foot Scrub

Ingredients

- ½ cup avocado (mashed)
- ¼ cup cornmeal
- 2 tablespoons avocado oil
- 1 tablespoon sea salt

Directions

1. In a bowl combine all the ingredients together
2. Apply to feet and scrub gently
3. Allow the scrub to stay on your feet for at least 10 minutes (longer if you have time)
4. Rinse off and dry your feet
5. Apply your favorite moisturizer and enjoy your smooth skin

Foot Soaks

There's nothing better than a good foot soak. You can create some amazing recipes that will leave your feet feeling as though they have been treated at a top boutique spa. Make these foot soaks and pamper your feet at home at least once a week. You owe it to yourself!

Decide ahead of time whether you want to be in front of the TV soaking your feet or whether you would prefer to relax alone in the tranquillity of your bathroom or bedroom. It's up to you so decide what works best at the time.

Minty Lime Foot Soak

Ingredients

- 1 cup Epsom salt
- ½ cup baking soda
- Zest of one lime
- 4 drops peppermint essential oil
- 1 teaspoon grated lime peel

Directions

1. Fill a foot spa or large basin with warm water
2. Add all the ingredients
3. Soak your feet for at least 15 minutes (or until the water gets cold)
4. Rinse off and dry your feet
5. Apply your favorite moisturizer and enjoy your lovely feet

Lemon Foot Odor Soak

Ingredients

- 1 cup Epsom salts
- 2 tablespoons baking soda
- 1 tablespoon grated lemon peel
- 6 drops lemon essential oil

Directions

1. Fill a foot spa or large basin with warm water
2. Add the Epsom salts, baking powder, lemon peel and essential oils
3. Mix until well blended
4. Soak your feet for at least 15 minutes (or until the water gets cold)
5. Rinse off and dry your feet
6. Apply your favorite moisturizer and enjoy your odor free feet

Magnificent Milk & Honey Foot Soak

Ingredients

- ¼ cup fresh lemon juice
- 2 tablespoons olive oil
- ¼ cup milk
- 3 tablespoons honey
- Pinch of cinnamon

Directions

1. Fill a foot spa or large basin with warm water
2. Add all the ingredients and mix until well blended
3. Soak your feet for at least 15 minutes (or until the water gets cold)
4. Rinse off and dry your feet
5. Apply your favorite moisturizer and enjoy your nice fresh feet

Luscious Lavender Foot Soak

Ingredients

- ¼ cup sea salt
- Handful of fresh lavender leaves
- 8 drops lavender essential oil

Directions

1. Fill a foot spa or large basin with warm water
2. Add all the ingredients and mix until well blended
3. Soak your feet for at least 15 minutes (or until the water gets cold)
4. Rinse off and dry your feet
5. Apply your favorite moisturizer and enjoy your nice lush feet

Rice Foot Soak

Ingredients

- ½ cup of rice (partially cooked with water remaining)
- 3 tablespoons baking soda
- 1 tablespoon parsley (chopped)

Directions

1. Half fill a foot spa or large basin with warm water
2. Add the rice with its water and the other ingredients and mix until well blended
3. Top up with a bit more water if needed
4. Soak your feet for at least 15 minutes (or until the water gets cold)
5. Rinse off and pat your feet dry
6. Apply your favorite moisturizer and enjoy your nice smooth skin

Really Rosy Foot Soak

Ingredients

- ½ cup Epsom salts
- ½ cup white sugar
- ¼ cup baking soda
- 2 tablespoons dried rose leaves
- 8 drops rose essential oil

Directions

1. Fill a foot spa or large basin with warm water
2. Add all the ingredients and mix until well blended
3. Soak your feet for at least 15 minutes (or until the water gets cold)
4. Rinse off and pat your feet dry
5. Apply your favorite moisturizer and enjoy your nice fresh feet

Emergency Foot Reviver

Ingredients

- ¼ cup jojoba oil
- 3 drops peppermint essential oil
- 3 drops grapefruit essential oil
- 3 drops sandalwood essential oil
- Pinch of Black pepper

Directions

1. Fill a foot spa or large basin with warm water
2. Add all the ingredients and mix until well blended
3. Soak your feet for at least 15 minutes (or until the water gets cold)
4. Rinse off and pat your feet dry
5. Apply your favorite moisturizer and enjoy your nice revived feet

Calming Chamomile Foot Soak

Ingredients

- 4 chamomile tea bags
- ½ cup Epsom salts
- 3 tablespoons honey

Directions

1. Fill a foot spa or large basin with warm water
2. Add all the ingredients and mix until well blended
3. Soak your feet for at least 15 minutes (or until the water gets cold)
4. Rinse off and pat your feet dry
5. Apply your favorite moisturizer and enjoy your rejuvenated feet

Olive Lemon Foot Soak

Ingredients

- 1 cup lemon juice
- 3 tablespoons olive oil
- ¼ cup milk
- ½ teaspoon grated lemon

Directions

1. Fill a foot spa or large basin with warm water
2. Add all the ingredients and mix until well blended
3. Soak your feet for at least 15 minutes (or until the water gets cold)
4. Rinse off and pat your feet dry
5. Apply your favorite moisturizer and enjoy your nice fresh feet

Orange Foot Soak

Ingredients

- ½ cup Epsom salts
- ½ cup baking soda
- 6 drops orange essential oil

Directions

1. Fill a foot spa or large basin with warm water
2. Add all the ingredients and mix until well blended
3. Soak your feet for at least 15 minutes (or until the water gets cold)
4. Rinse off and pat your feet dry
5. Apply your favorite moisturizer and enjoy your nice fresh feet

Apple Cider Vinegar Foot Soak

Ingredients

- 2 cups Apple Cider Vinegar
- ½ cup Epsom salt
- 5 drops eucalyptus essential oil
- 4 drops lemon essential oil

Directions

1. Fill a foot spa or large basin with warm water
2. Add all the ingredients and mix until well blended
3. Soak your feet for at least 15 minutes (or until the water gets cold)
4. Rinse off and pat your feet dry
5. Apply your favorite moisturizer and enjoy your nice fresh feet

Easy Eucalyptus Foot Soak

Ingredients

- ¼ cup sea salt
- 5 drops eucalyptus essential oil
- 2 tablespoons fresh mint (chopped)

Directions

1. Fill a foot spa or large basin with warm water
2. Add all the ingredients and mix until well blended
3. Soak your feet for at least 15 minutes (or until the water gets cold)
4. Rinse off and pat your feet dry
5. Apply your favorite moisturizer and enjoy your nice fresh feet

Forget Fungus Foot Soak

Ingredients

- ¼ cup apple cider vinegar
- 2 tablespoons baking soda
- 5 drops tea tree oil
- 5 drops lavender oil

Directions

1. Fill a foot spa or large basin with warm water
2. Add all the ingredients and mix until well blended
3. Soak your feet for at least 15 minutes (or until the water gets cold)
4. Rinse off and pat your feet dry
5. Apply your favorite moisturizer and enjoy your nice clean feet

Aching Feet Foot Soak

Ingredients

- 3 drops rosemary essential oil
- 2 tablespoon fresh rosemary (finely chopped)
- 2 drops tea tree essential oil
- 1 tablespoon baking soda

Directions

1. Fill a foot spa or large basin with warm water
2. Add all the ingredients and mix until well blended
3. Soak your feet for at least 15 minutes (or until the water gets cold)
4. Rinse off and pat your feet dry
5. Apply your favorite moisturizer and enjoy your nice renewed feet

Super Sore Foot Soak

Ingredients

- ¼ cup milk
- 3 drops peppermint essential oil
- 3 drops chamomile essential oil
- 3 drops lavender essential oil
- Pinch of cinnamon

Directions

1. Fill a foot spa or large basin with warm water
2. Add all the ingredients and mix until well blended
3. Soak your feet for at least 15 minutes (or until the water gets cold)
4. Rinse off and pat your feet dry
5. Apply your favorite moisturizer and enjoy your gentle fresh skin

Orange & Ginger Foot Soak

Ingredients

- ¼ cup jojoba oil
- 1 inch piece of ginger (grated)
- 1 teaspoon cayenne pepper
- ¼ cup brown sugar
- 4 drops orange essential oil

Directions

1. Fill a foot spa or large basin with warm water
2. Add all the ingredients and mix until well blended
3. Soak your feet for at least 15 minutes (or until the water gets cold)
4. Rinse off and pat your feet dry
5. Apply your favorite moisturizer and enjoy your nicely relaxed feet

Dead Sea Salts Soak

Ingredients

- 2 cups dead sea salt
- Handful of fresh lavender leaves
- 4 drops lemon essential oil
- 1 teaspoon baking soda

Directions

1. Fill a foot spa or large basin with warm water
2. Add all the ingredients and mix until well blended
3. Soak your feet for at least 15 minutes (or until the water gets cold)
4. Rinse off and pat your feet dry
5. Apply your favorite moisturizer and enjoy your nicely rejuvenated feet

Jasmine Foot Soak

Ingredients

- 1 cup dried Jasmine flowers
- 3 drops sandalwood essential oil
- 2 tablespoons olive oil

Directions

1. Fill a foot spa or large basin with warm water
2. Add all the ingredients and mix until well blended
3. Soak your feet for at least 15 minutes (or until the water gets cold)
4. Rinse off and pat your feet dry
5. Apply your favorite moisturizer and enjoy your nice fresh feet

Pumpkin Foot Soak

Ingredients

- 2 pumpkin tea bags
- 2 cinnamon tea bags
- Handful of fresh pumpkin seeds

Directions

1. Fill a foot spa or large basin with warm water
2. Add the teabags and allow to brew
3. Next, add the pumpkin seeds
4. Soak your feet for at least 15 minutes (or until the water gets cold)
5. Rinse off and pat your feet dry
6. Apply your favorite moisturizer and enjoy your nicely cared for feet

Grapefruit & Lime Foot Soak

Ingredients

- 1 cup sea salt
- 1 grapefruit (sliced)
- 1 lime (sliced)
- 3 drops lime essential oil
- 3 drops grapefruit essential oil
- ½ teaspoon brown sugar

Directions

1. Fill a foot spa or large basin with warm water
2. Add all the ingredients and mix until well blended
3. Soak your feet for at least 15 minutes (or until the water gets cold)
4. Rinse off and pat your feet dry
5. Apply your favorite moisturizer and enjoy your tip top feet

Smelly Feet Foot Soak

Ingredients

- Juice of 1 lemon
- 3 drops cypress essential oil
- 2 drops of sage essential oil
- 2 drops lime essential oil

Directions

1. Fill a foot spa or large basin with warm water
2. Add all the ingredients and mix until well blended
3. Soak your feet for at least 15 minutes (or until the water gets cold)
4. Rinse off and pat your feet dry
5. Apply your favorite moisturizer and enjoy your nice fresh feet

Dead Tired Foot Soak

Ingredients

- 1 cup dead sea salt
- 2 tablespoons lavender oil
- 3 drops lavender essential oil
- 3 drops tea tree essential oil

Directions

1. Fill a foot spa or large basin with warm water
2. Add all the ingredients and mix until well blended
3. Soak your feet for at least 15 minutes (or until the water gets cold)
4. Rinse off and pat your feet dry
5. Apply your favorite moisturizer and enjoy your nicely cared for feet

Sweet Cucumber Foot Soak

Ingredients

- ½ cucumber (chopped and mashed)
- 2 tablespoons baking soda
- ½ cup brown sugar
- 3 drops lemon essential oil

Directions

1. Fill a foot spa or large basin with warm water
2. Add all the ingredients and mix until well blended
3. Soak your feet for at least 15 minutes (or until the water gets cold)
4. Rinse off and pat your feet dry
5. Apply your favorite moisturizer and enjoy your replenished skin

Heel Balms

You are on your feet a lot and your heels can often go without the full treatment they deserve. Your skin can get rough on your heels, especially in winter so you need to make sure you keep them properly moisturized. Make and apply these heel balms for optimum heel care.

Rich Coco Heel Balm

Ingredients

- 2 oz. coconut oil
- 1 ½ oz. avocado oil
- 1 oz. cocoa butter
- 1 oz. castor oil
- 1 oz. shea butter

Directions

1. In a large bowl, mix the coconut oil, avocado oil and castor oil together
2. Heat a small pan of water and add a glass bowl to it
3. Put the shea butter and cocoa butter in the glass bowl and allow the butters to melt together
4. Pour the oil mixture into the butters and mix well
5. Pour the mixture into a sterilized container and allow it to cool before using it
6. When ready wash your feet and apply the balm to your heels
7. Rub in gently for a good few minutes making sure you moisturize your heels thoroughly
8. Apply morning and night for best results

Cinnamon & Orange Heel Balm

Ingredients

- 200ml Super Aqueous Cream
- 50ml glycerine
- 1 oz. shea butter
- 1 oz. cocoa butter
- 1 teaspoon cinnamon
- 5 drops orange essential oil

Directions

1. Heat a small pan of water and add a glass bowl to it
2. Put all the ingredients in the glass bowl and allow the butters, oil and cream to melt together
3. Pour the mixture into a sterilized container and allow it to cool and harden slightly
4. Add the essential oil
5. When ready wash your feet and apply the balm to your heels
6. Rub in gently for a good few minutes making sure you moisturize your heels thoroughly
7. Apply morning and night for best results

Neem Oil Heel Balm

Ingredients

- 200ml coconut oil
- 200ml sweet almond oil
- 100g soy wax
- 200ml Neem oil

Directions

1. Heat a small pan of water and add a glass bowl to it
2. Put all the ingredients in the bowl and melt until blended together
3. Pour the mixture into a sterilized container and allow it to cool before using it
4. When ready wash your feet and apply the balm to your heels
5. Rub in gently for a good few minutes making sure you moisturize your heels thoroughly
6. Apply morning and night for best results

Jojoba Heel Balm

Ingredients

- 3 tablespoons cocoa butter
- 2 tablespoons beeswax
- ¼ cup sweet almond oil

Directions

1. Heat a small pan of water and add a glass bowl to it
2. Put all the ingredients in the bowl and allow the ingredients to melt together
3. Pour the mixture into a sterilized container and allow it to cool before using it
4. When ready wash your feet and apply the balm to your heels
5. Rub in gently for a good few minutes making sure you moisturize your heels thoroughly
6. Apply morning and night for best results

Emu Oil Heel Balm

Ingredients

- 6 teaspoons emu oil
- 1 teaspoon lanolin
- 2 teaspoons shea butter
- 2 teaspoons beeswax
- 7 drops ylang ylang essential oil
- 10 drops orange essential oil
- 1 ½ oz. avocado oil
- 1 oz. cocoa butter
- 1 oz. castor oil
- 1 oz. shea butter

Directions

1. Heat a small pan of water and add a glass bowl to it
2. Put all the ingredients (except the essential oils) in the bowl and allow everything to melt together
3. Allow to cool slightly and add the essential oils
4. Pour the mixture into a sterilized container and allow it to cool before using it
5. When ready wash your feet and apply the balm to your heels
6. Rub in gently for a good few minutes making sure you moisturize your heels thoroughly
7. Apply morning and night for best results

Lavender Heel Balm

Ingredients

- ¼ cup coconut oil
- 5 drops vitamin E oil
- 2 tablespoons beeswax
- 2 tablespoons shea butter
- 2 tablespoons dried lavender leaves
- 3 drops lavender essential oil

Directions

1. Heat a small pan of water and add a glass bowl to it
2. Put all the ingredients (except the essential oils) in the bowl and allow everything to melt together
3. Allow to cool slightly and add the essential oils
4. Pour the mixture into a sterilized container and allow it to cool before using it
5. When ready wash your feet and apply the balm to your heels
6. Rub in gently for a good few minutes making sure you moisturize your heels thoroughly
7. Apply morning and night for best results

Honey Orange Heel Balm

Ingredients

- 1 cup honey
- 1-2 tablespoons milk
- Juice of half an orange

Directions

1. Warm the honey for 10-15 seconds in the microwave to make it more spreadable
2. Add the milk to the honey as well as the orange juice
3. Pour the mixture into a sterilized container
4. When ready wash your feet and apply the balm to your heels
5. Relax and leave it to soak into your heels for at least 20 minutes
6. Rinse off and pat your feet dry
7. Apply morning and night for best results

Organic Olive Oil Heel Balm

Ingredients

- 2 tablespoons organic olive oil
- 2 tablespoons avocado oil
- 3 drops tea tree oil

Directions

1. Heat a small pan of water and add a glass bowl to it
2. Put all the ingredients (except the essential oils) in the bowl and allow everything to melt together
3. Allow to cool slightly and add the essential oils
4. Pour the mixture into a sterilized container and allow it to cool before using it
5. When ready wash your feet and apply the balm to your heels
6. Rub in gently for a good few minutes making sure you moisturize your heels thoroughly
7. Apply morning and night for best results

Shea & Lemongrass Heel Balm

Ingredients

- 1 tablespoon jojoba oil
- 1 tablespoon avocado oil
- 1 tablespoon shea butter
- 6 drops lemongrass essential oil

Directions

1. Heat a small pan of water and add a glass bowl to it
2. Put all the ingredients (except the essential oil) in the bowl and allow everything to melt together
3. Allow to cool slightly and add the essential oils
4. Pour the mixture into a sterilized container and allow it to cool before using it
5. When ready wash your feet and apply the balm to your heels
6. Rub in gently for a good few minutes making sure you moisturize your heels thoroughly
7. Apply morning and night for best results

Tea Tree Heel Balm

Ingredients

- 2 tablespoons shea butter
- 2 tablespoons coconut oil
- 2 tablespoons olive oil
- 10 drops vanilla essential oil
- 5 drops peppermint essential oil
- ½ oz. beeswax

Directions

1. Heat a small pan of water and add a glass bowl to it
2. Put all the ingredients (except the essential oils) in the bowl and allow everything to melt together
3. Allow to cool slightly and add the essential oils
4. Pour the mixture into a sterilized container and allow it to cool before using it
5. When ready wash your feet and apply the balm to your heels
6. Rub in gently for a good few minutes making sure you moisturize your heels thoroughly
7. Apply morning and night for best results

Conclusion

Well there you have it, 48 of my best foot care recipes. They each offer great amounts of cleaning, exfoliating, detoxifying and moisturizing benefits.

You really owe it to your feet to treat them well. Your feet need to carry you around today and hopefully for years to come so by adopting a good foot care routine, your feet will feel better and you will feel better overall.

I do hope you enjoy making and using the recipes in this book as much as I did putting it together for you. I wish you very happy foot care.

Lorraine Xx

Don't forget to check out my other book in this series, all available on Amazon

- Homemade Lotions: 41 All Natural, Simple & Easy To Make Body Lotions, Body Butters & Lotion Bars
- How To Make Bath Bombs: *Bath Salts & Bubble Baths: 53 All Natural & Organic Recipes*
- Homemade Beauty Products : Over 50 All Natural Recipes For Face Masks, Facial Cleansers & Face Creams: Natural Organic Recipes For Youthful Skin
- Homemade Body Scrubs : 52 All Natural, Simple & Easy To Make Body Scrubs, Face Masks, Lip Balms & Body Washes: Amazing DIY Organic & Healing Scrubs To Renew Your Skin & Reverse The Signs Of Aging

Made in the USA
Las Vegas, NV
04 May 2023

71580561R00036